Air Fryer Delights

An Unmissable Recipe Collection for Your Air Fryer Meals

Eva Sheppard

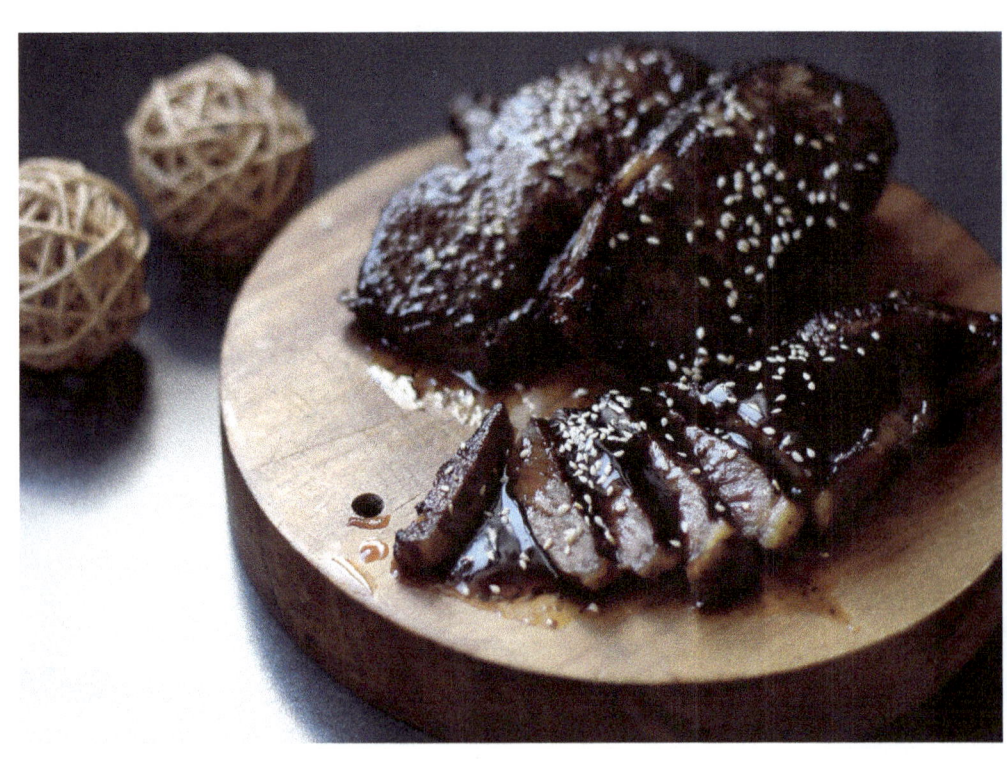

© **Copyright 2021 - All rights reserved.**

The content contained within this book may not be reproduced, duplicated or transmitted without direct written permission from the author or the publisher.

Under no circumstances will any blame or legal responsibility be held against the publisher, or author, for any damages, reparation, or monetary loss due to the information contained within this book. Either directly or indirectly.

Legal Notice:

This book is copyright protected. This book is only for personal use. You cannot amend, distribute, sell, use, quote or paraphrase any part, or the content within this book, without the consent of the author or publisher.

Disclaimer Notice:

Please note the information contained within this document is for educational and entertainment purposes only. All effort has been executed to present accurate, up to date, and reliable, complete information. No warranties of any kind are declared or implied. Readers acknowledge that the author is not engaging in the rendering of legal, financial, medical or professional advice. The content within this book has been derived from various sources. Please consult a licensed professional before attempting any techniques outlined in this book.

By reading this document, the reader agrees that under no circumstances is the author responsible for any losses, direct or indirect, which are incurred as a result of the use of information contained within this document, including, but not limited to, — errors, omissions, or inaccuracies.

TABLE OF CONTENT

Lentils Snack *8*
Air Fried Corn *10*
Salmon Tarts *11*
Parmesan Crusted Pickles *14*
Breaded Mushrooms *16*
Cheesy Sticks with Sweet Thai Sauce... *18*
Bacon Wrapped Avocados *20*
Hot Chicken Wingettes *23*
Bacon & Chicken Wrapped Jalapenos *25*
Mouth-Watering Salami Sticks *28*
Carrot Crisps *30*
Calamari with Olives *31*
Sweet Mixed Nuts *33*
Cheesy Onion Rings *35*
Cheesy Sausage Balls... *37*
Crusted Coconut Shrimp *40*
Quick Cheese Sticks *42*
Spicy Cheese Lings... *43*
Radish Chips... *45*
Zucchini Parmesan Chips *48*

Paprika Chicken Nuggets *50*

Cool Chicken Croquettes *52*

Herbed Croutons With Brie Cheese *55*

Cheesy Bacon Fries *56*

Oriental Grilled Family Steak *58*

Tandoori Spiced Sirloin *61*

Ribeye Steak with Peaches *63*

Kansas City Ribs *65*

Grilled Steak Cubes with Charred Onions *67*

Trip Tip Roast with Grilled Avocado *69*

Bourbon Grilled Beef *71*

Paprika Beef Flank Steak *73*

Espresso-Rubbed Steak *75*

New York Beef Strips *77*

Smoked Beef Chuck *80*

Sous Vide Smoked Brisket *83*

Skirt Steak with Mojo Marinade *85*

Dijon-Marinated Skirt Steak *87*

Grilled Carne Asada Steak *89*

Chimichurri-Style Steak *91*

Strip Steak with Cucumber Yogurt Sauce *93*

Pork Bites *95*

Banana Chips *97*

Lemony Apple Bites *98*

Zucchini Balls *99*

Basil and Cilantro Crackers ***101***
Balsamic Zucchini Slices ***104***
Turmeric Carrot Chips ***105***
Chives Radish Snack ***106***

Lentils Snack

Preparation time: 5 minutes

Cooking time: 12 minutes

Servings: 4

Ingredients:

- 15 ounces canned lentils, drained
- ½ teaspoon cumin, ground
- 1 tablespoon olive oil
- 1 teaspoon sweet paprika
- Salt and black pepper to taste

Directions:

1. Place all ingredients in a bowl and mix well.
2. Transfer the mixture to your air fryer and cook at 400 degrees F for 12 minutes.
3. Divide into bowls and serve as a snack -or a side, or appetizer!.

Nutrition Values: calories 151, fat 1, fiber 6, carbs 10, protein 6

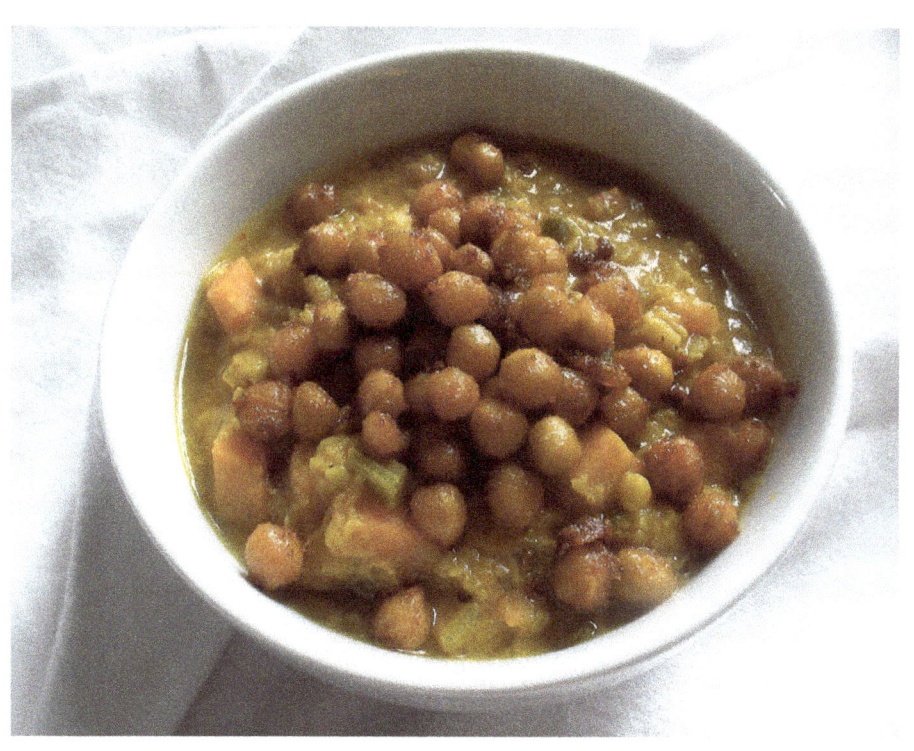

Air Fried Corn

Preparation time: 5 minutes

Cooking time: 10 minutes

Servings: 4

Ingredients:

- 2 tablespoons corn kernels
- 2½ tablespoons butter

Directions:

1. In a pan that fits your air fryer, mix the corn with the butter.
2. Place the pan in the fryer and cook at 400 degrees F for 10 minutes.
3. Serve as a snack and enjoy!

Nutrition Values: calories 70, fat 2, fiber 2, carbs 7, protein 3

Salmon Tarts

Preparation Time: 20 min

Servings: 15

Nutrition Values: Calories: 415; Carbs: 43g; Fat: 23g; Protein: 10g

Ingredients

- 15 mini tart cases
- 4 eggs, lightly beaten
- ½ cup heavy cream
- Salt and black pepper
- 3 oz smoked salmon
- 6 oz cream cheese, divided into 15 pieces
- 6 fresh dill

Directions

1. Mix together eggs and cream in a pourable measuring container. Arrange the tarts into the air fryer. Pour in mixture into the tarts, about halfway up the side and top with a piece of salmon and a piece of cheese. Cook

for 10 minutes at 340 F, regularly check to avoid overcooking. Sprinkle dill and serve chilled.

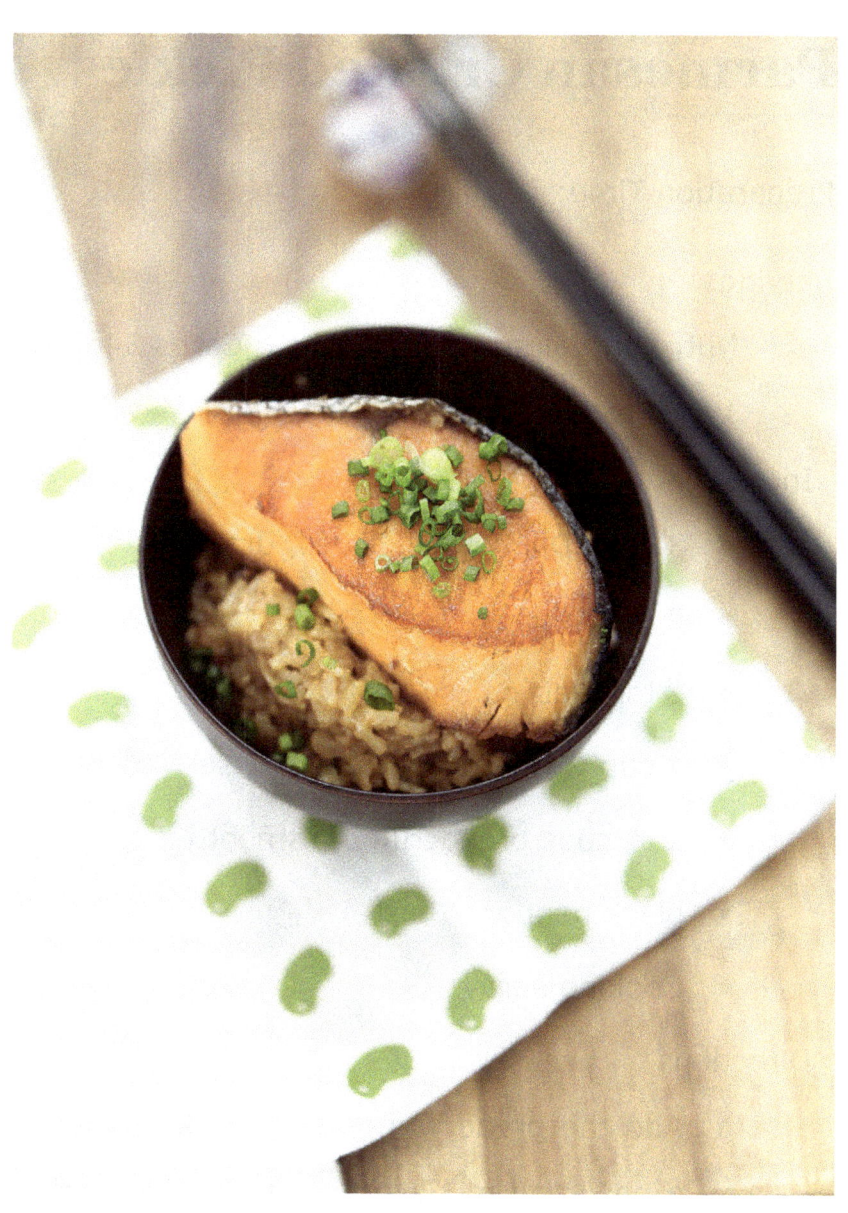

Parmesan Crusted Pickles

Preparation Time: 35 min

Servings: 4

Nutrition Values: Calories 335; Carbs 34g; Fat 14g; Protein 17g

Ingredients

- 3 cups Dill Pickles, sliced, drained
- 2 eggs
- 2 tsp water
- 1 cup Grated Parmesan cheese
- 1 ½ cups breadcrumbs, smooth
- black pepper to taste
- Cooking spray

Directions

1. Add the breadcrumbs and black pepper to a bowl and mix well; set aside. In another bowl, crack the eggs and beat with the water. Set aside. Add the cheese to a

separate bowl; set aside. Preheat the Air Fryer to 400 F.

2. Pull out the fryer basket and spray it lightly with cooking spray. Dredge the pickle slices it in the egg mixture, then in breadcrumbs and then in cheese. Place them in the fryer without overlapping.

3. Slide the fryer basket back in and cook for 4 minutes. Turn them and cook for further for 5 minutes, until crispy. Serve with a cheese dip.

Breaded Mushrooms

Preparation Time: 55 min

Servings: 4

Nutrition Values: Calories 487; Carbs 49g; Fat 22g; Protein 31g

Ingredients

- 1 lb small Button mushrooms, cleaned
- 2 cups breadcrumbs
- 2 eggs, beaten
- Salt and pepper to taste
- 2 cups Parmigiano Reggiano cheese, grated

Directions

1. Preheat the Air Fryer to 360 F. Pour the breadcrumbs in a bowl, add salt and pepper and mix well. Pour the cheese in a separate bowl and set aside. Dip each mushroom in the eggs, then in the crumbs, and then in the cheese.

2. Slide out the fryer basket and add 6 to 10 mushrooms. Cook them for 20 minutes, in batches, if needed. Serve with cheese dip.

Cheesy Sticks with Sweet Thai Sauce

Preparation Time: 2 hrs 20 min

Servings: 4

Nutrition Values: Calories 158; Carbs 14g; Fat 7g; Protein 9g

Ingredients

- 12 mozzarella string cheese
- 2 cups breadcrumbs
- 3 eggs
- 1 cup sweet thai sauce
- 4 tbsp skimmed milk

Directions

1. Pour the crumbs in a medium bowl. Crack the eggs into another bowl and beat with the milk. One after the other, dip each cheese sticks in the egg mixture, in the

crumbs, then egg mixture again and then in the crumbs again.

2. Place the coated cheese sticks on a cookie sheet and freeze for 1 to 2 hours. Preheat the Air Fryer to 380 F. Arrange the sticks in the fryer without overcrowding. Cook for 5 minutes, flipping them halfway through cooking to brown evenly. Cook in batches. Serve with a sweet thai sauce.

Bacon Wrapped Avocados

Preparation Time: 40 min

Servings: 6

Nutrition Values: Calories 193; Carbs 10g; Fat 16g; Protein 4g

Ingredients

- 12 thick strips bacon
- 3 large avocados, sliced
- ⅓ tsp salt
- ⅓ tsp chili powder
- ⅓ tsp cumin powder

Directions

1. Stretch the bacon strips to elongate and use a knife to cut in half to make 24 pieces. Wrap each bacon piece around a slice of avocado from one end to the other end. Tuck the end of bacon into the wrap. Arrange on a flat surface and season with salt, chili and cumin on both sides.

2. Arrange 4 to 8 wrapped pieces in the fryer and cook at 350 F for 8 minutes, or until the bacon is browned and crunchy, flipping halfway through to cook evenly. Remove onto a wire rack and repeat the process for the remaining avocado pieces.

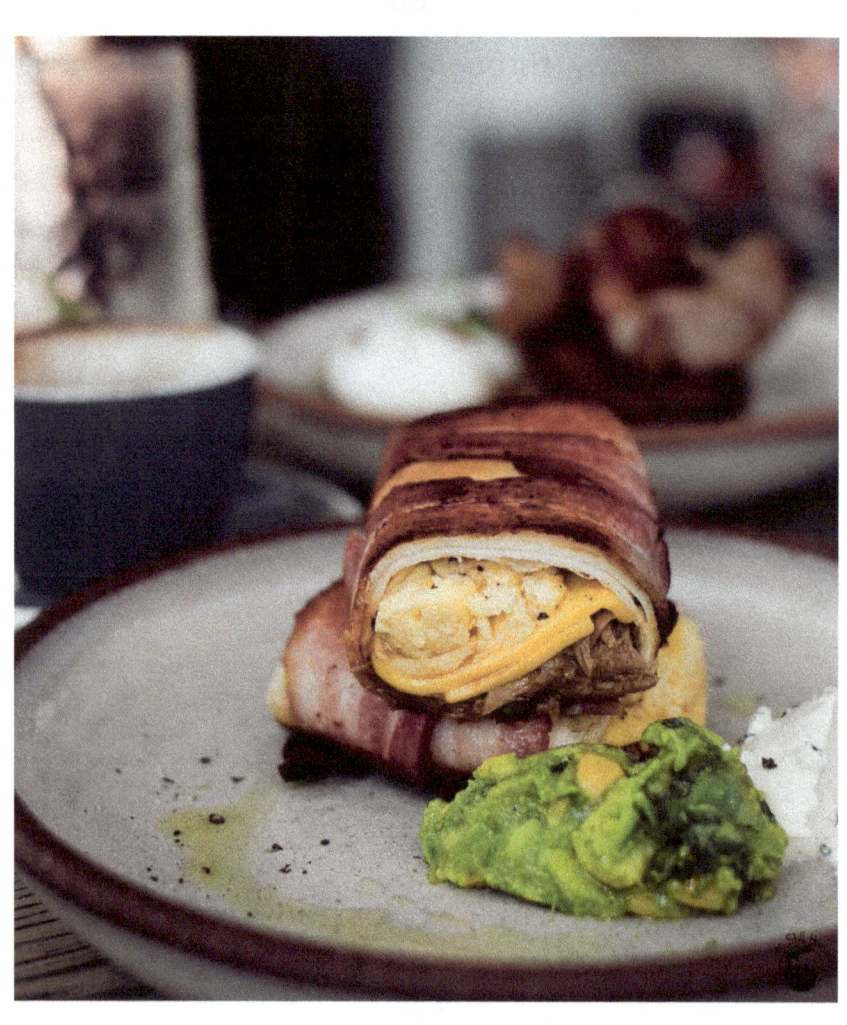

Hot Chicken Wingettes

Preparation Time: 45 min

Servings: 3

Nutrition Values: Calories 563; Carbs 2g; Fat 28g; Protein 35g

Ingredients

- 15 chicken wingettes
- Salt and pepper to taste
- ⅓ cup hot sauce
- ⅓ cup butter
- ½ tbsp vinegar

Directions

1. Preheat the Air Fryer to 360 F. Season the wingettes with pepper and salt. Add them to the air fryer and cook for 35 minutes. Toss every 5 minutes. Once ready, remove them into a bowl. Over low heat, melt the butter in a saucepan. Add the vinegar and hot sauce. Stir and cook for a minute.

2. Turn the heat off. Pour the sauce over the chicken. Toss to coat well. Transfer the chicken to a serving platter. Serve with a side of celery strips and blue cheese dressing.

Bacon & Chicken Wrapped Jalapenos

Preparation Time: 40 min

Servings: 4

Nutrition Values: Calories 244; Carbs 13g; Fat 12.8g; Protein 9.3g

Ingredients

- 8 Jalapeno peppers, halved lengthwise and seeded
- 4 chicken breasts, butterflied and halved
- 6 oz cream cheese
- 6 oz Cheddar cheese
- 16 slices bacon
- 1 cup breadcrumbs
- Salt and pepper to taste
- 2 eggs
- Cooking spray

Directions

1. Season the chicken with pepper and salt on both sides. In a bowl, add cream cheese, cheddar, a pinch of pepper and salt. Mix well. Take each jalapeno and spoon in the cheese mixture to the brim. On a working board, flatten each piece of chicken and lay 2 bacon slices each on them. Place a stuffed jalapeno on each laid out chicken and bacon set, and wrap the jalapenos in them.

2. Preheat the air fryer to 350 F. Add the eggs to a bowl and pour the breadcrumbs in another bowl. Also, set a flat plate aside. Take each wrapped jalapeno and dip it into the eggs and then in the breadcrumbs. Place them on the flat plate. Lightly grease the fryer basket with cooking spray. Arrange 4-5 breaded jalapenos in the basket, and cook for 7 minutes.

3. Prepare a paper towel lined plate; set aside. Once the timer beeps, open the fryer, turn

the jalapenos, and cook further for 4 minutes. Once ready, remove them onto the paper towel lined plate. Repeat the cooking process for the remaining jalapenos. Serve with a sweet dip for an enhanced taste.

Mouth-Watering Salami Sticks

Preparation Time: 2 hrs 10 min

Servings: 3

Nutrition Values: Calories 428; Carbs 12g; Fat 16g; Protein 42g

Ingredients

- 1 lb ground beef
- 3 tbsp sugar
- A pinch garlic powder
- A pinch chili powder
- Salt to taste
- 1 tsp liquid smoke

Directions

1. Place the meat, sugar, garlic powder, chili powder, salt and liquid smoke in a bowl. Mix with a spoon. Mold out 4 sticks with your hands, place them on a plate, and

refrigerate for 2 hours. Cook at 350 F. for 10 minutes, flipping once halfway through.

Carrot Crisps

Preparation Time: 20 min

Servings: 2

Nutrition Values: Calories 35; Carbs 8g; Fat 3g; Protein 1g

Ingredients

- 3 large carrots, washed and peeled
- Salt to taste
- Cooking spray

Directions

2. Using a mandolin slicer, slice the carrots very thinly heightwise. Put the carrot strips in a bowl and season with salt to taste. Grease the fryer basket lightly with cooking spray, and add the carrot strips. Cook at 350 F for 10 minutes, stirring once halfway through.

Calamari with Olives

Preparation Time: 25 min

Servings: 3

Nutrition Values: Calories 128; Carbs 0g; Fat 3g; Protein 22g

Ingredients

- ½ lb calamari rings
- ½ piece coriander, chopped
- 2 strips chili pepper, chopped
- 1 tbsp olive oil
- 1 cup pimiento-stuffed green olives, sliced
- Salt and black pepper to taste

Directions

1. In a bowl, add rings, chili pepper, salt, black pepper, oil, and coriander. Mix and let marinate for 10 minutes. Pour the calamari into an oven-safe bowl, that fits into the fryer basket.

2. Slide the fryer basket out, place the bowl in it, and slide the basket back in. Cook for 15 minutes stirring every 5 minutes using a spoon, at 400 F. After 15 minutes, and add in the olives.
3. Stir, close and continue to cook for 3 minutes. Once ready, transfer to a serving platter. Serve warm with a side of bread slices and mayonnaise.

Sweet Mixed Nuts

Preparation Time: 25 min

Servings: 5

Nutrition Values: Calories 147; Carbs 10g; Fat 12g; Protein 3g

Ingredients

- ½ cup pecans
- ½ cup walnuts
- ½ cup almonds
- A pinch cayenne pepper
- 2 tbsp sugar
- 2 tbsp egg whites
- 2 tsp cinnamon
- Cooking spray

Directions

1. Add the pepper, sugar, and cinnamon to a bowl and mix well; set aside. In another bowl, mix in the pecans, walnuts, almonds, and egg whites. Add the spice mixture to

the nuts and give it a good mix. Lightly grease the fryer basket with cooking spray.

2. Pour in the nuts, and cook them for 10 minutes. Stir the nuts using a wooden vessel, and cook for further for 10 minutes. Pour the nuts in the bowl. Let cool before crunching on them.

Cheesy Onion Rings

Preparation Time: 20 min

Servings: 3

Nutrition Values: Calories 205; Carbs 14g; Fat 11g; Protein 12g

Ingredients

- 1 onion, peeled and sliced into 1-inch rings
- ¾ cup Parmesan cheese
- 2 medium eggs, beaten
- 1 tsp garlic powder
- A pinch of salt
- 1 cup flour
- 1 tsp paprika powder

Directions

1. Add the eggs to a bowl; set aside In another bowl, add cheese, garlic powder, salt, flour, and paprika. Mix with a spoon. Dip each onion ring in egg, then in the cheese

mixture, in the egg again and finally in the cheese mixture.

2. Add the rings to the basket and cook them for 8 minutes at 350 F. Remove onto a serving platter and serve with a cheese or tomatoes dip.

Cheesy Sausage Balls

Preparation Time: 50 min

Servings: 8

Nutrition Values: Calories 456; Carbs 23g; Fat 36g; Protein 36g

Ingredients

- 1 ½ lb ground sausages
- 2 ¼ cups Cheddar cheese, shredded
- 1 ½ cup flour
- ¾ tsp baking soda
- 4 eggs
- ¾ cup sour cream
- 1 tsp dried oregano
- 1 tsp smoked paprika
- 2 tsp garlic powder
- ½ cup liquid coconut oil

Directions

1. In a pan over medium heat, add the sausages and brown for 3-4 minutes. Drain the excess fat and set aside. In a bowl, sift in baking soda, and flour. Set aside. In another bowl, add eggs, sour cream, oregano, paprika, coconut oil, and garlic powder. Whisk to combine well. Combine the egg and flour mixtures using a spatula.

2. Add the cheese and sausages. Fold in and let it sit for 5 minutes to thicken. Rub your hands with coconut oil and mold out bite-size balls out of the batter. Place them on a tray, and refrigerate for 15 minutes. Then, add them in the air fryer, without overcrowding. Cook for 10 minutes per round, at 400 F, in batches if needed.

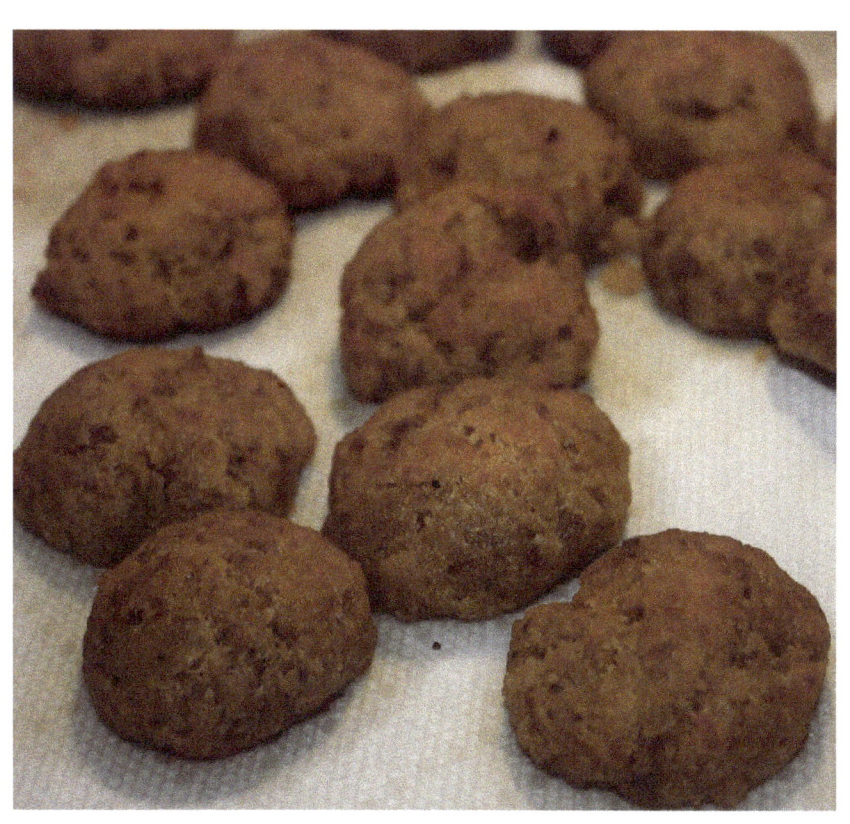

Crusted Coconut Shrimp

Preparation Time: 30 min

Servings: 5

Nutrition Values: Calories 149; Carbs 7g; Fat 2g; Protein 18g

Ingredients

- 1 lb jumbo shrimp, peeled and deveined
- ¾ cup shredded coconut
- 1 tbsp maple syrup
- ½ cup breadcrumbs
- ⅓ cup cornstarch
- ½ cup milk

Directions

1. Pour the cornstarch in a zipper bag, add shrimp, zip the bag up and shake vigorously to coat with the cornstarch. Mix the syrup and milk in a bowl and set aside. In a separate bowl, mix the breadcrumbs and shredded coconut. Open the zipper bag

and remove each shrimp while shaking off excess starch.

2. Dip each shrimp in the milk mixture and then in the crumbs mixture while pressing loosely to trap enough crumbs and coconut. Place the coated shrimp in the fryer without overcrowding. Cook 12 minutes at 350 F, flipping once halfway through. Cook until golden brown. Serve with a coconut based dip.

Quick Cheese Sticks

Preparation Time: 5 min

Servings: 12

Nutrition Values: Calories 256; Carbs 8g; Fat 21g; Protein 16g

Ingredients

- 6 -6 ozbread cheese
- 2 tbsp butter
- 2 cups panko crumbs

Directions

1. Put the butter in a bowl and melt in the microwave, for 2 minutes; set aside. With a knife, cut the cheese into equal sized sticks. Brush each stick with butter and dip into panko crumbs. Arrange the cheese sticks in a single layer on the fryer basket. Cook at 390 F for 10 minutes. Flip them halfway through, to brown evenly; serve warm.

Spicy Cheese Lings

Preparation Time: 25 min

Servings: 3

Nutrition Values: Calories 225; Carbs 35g; Fat 5.6g; Protein 8g

Ingredients

- 4 tbsp grated cheese + extra for rolling
- 1 cup flour + extra for kneading
- ¼ tsp chili powder
- ½ tsp baking powder
- 3 tsp butter
- A pinch of salt
- Water

Directions

1. In a bowl, mix in the cheese, flour, baking powder, chili powder, butter, and salt. The mixture should be crusty. Add some drops of water and mix well to get a dough. Remove the dough on a flat surface.

2. Rub some extra flour in your palms and on the surface, and knead the dough for a while. Using a rolling pin, roll the dough out into a thin sheet. With a pastry cutter, cut the dough into your desired lings' shape. Add the cheese lings in the basket, and cook for 6 minutes at 350 F, flipping once halfway through.

Radish Chips

Preparation Time: 30 min

Servings: 4

Nutrition Values: Calories 25; Carbs 0.2g; Fat 2g; Protein 0.1g

Ingredients

- 10 radishes, leaves removed and cleaned
- Salt to season
- Water
- Cooking spray

Directions

1. Using a mandolin, slice the radishes thinly. Place them in a pot and cover them with water. Heat the pot on a stovetop, and bring to boil, until the radishes are translucent, for 4 minutes. After 4 minutes, drain the radishes through a sieve; set aside. Grease the fryer basket with cooking spray.

2. Add in the radish slices and cook for 8 minutes, flipping once halfway through. Cook until golden brown, at 400 F. Meanwhile, prepare a paper towel-lined plate. Once the radishes are ready, transfer them to the paper towel-lined plate. Season with salt, and serve with ketchup or garlic mayo.

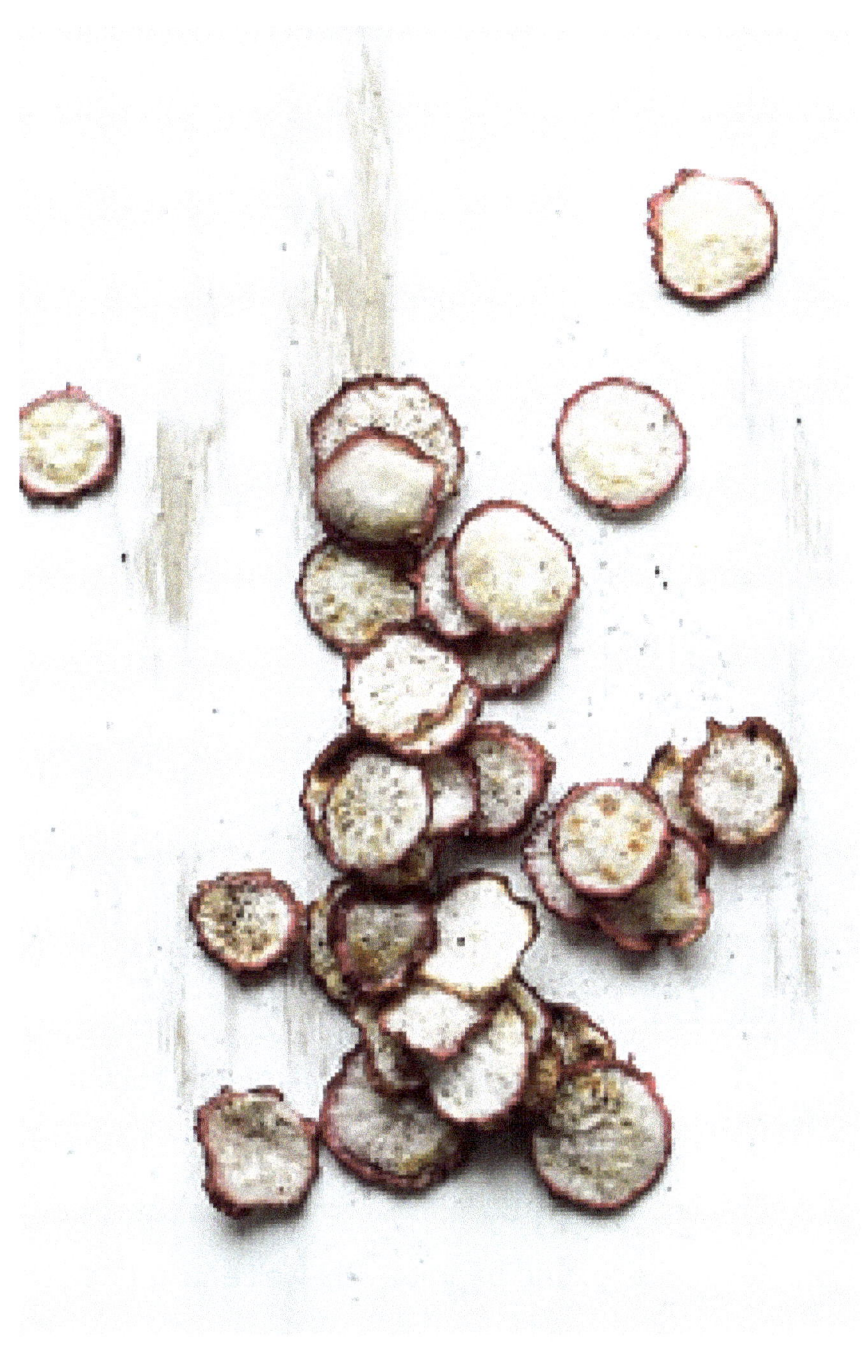

Zucchini Parmesan Chips

Preparation Time: 20 min

Servings: 3

Nutrition Values: Calories 268; Carbs 13g; Fat 16g; Protein 17g

Ingredients

- 3 medium zucchinis
- 1 cup breadcrumbs
- 2 eggs, beaten
- 1 cup grated Parmesan cheese
- Salt and pepper to taste
- 1 tsp smoked paprika
- Cooking spray

Directions

1. With a mandolin cutter, slice the zucchinis thinly. Use paper towels to press out excess liquid. In a bowl, add crumbs, salt, pepper, cheese, and paprika. Mix well and set aside. Set a wire rack or tray aside. Dip each

zucchini slice in egg and then in the cheese mix while pressing to coat them well.

2. Place them on the wire rack. Spray the coated slices with oil. Put the slices in the fryer basket in a single layer without overlapping. Cook at 350 F for 8 minutes for each batch. Serve sprinkled with salt and with a spicy dip.

Paprika Chicken Nuggets

Preparation Time: 1 hr 20 min

Servings: 4

Nutrition Values: Calories 548; Carbs 51g; Fat 23g; Protein 49g

Ingredients

- 2 chicken breasts, bones removed
- 2 tbsp paprika
- 2 cups milk
- 2 eggs
- 4 tsp onion powder
- 1 ½ tsp garlic powder
- Salt and pepper to taste
- 1 cups flour
- 2 cups breadcrumbs
- Cooking spray

Directions

1. Cut the chicken into 1-inch chunks. In a bowl, mix in paprika, onion, garlic, salt, pepper, flour, and breadcrumbs. In another bowl, crack the eggs, add the milk and beat them together. Prepare a tray. Dip each chicken chunk in the egg mixture, place them on the tray, and refrigerate for 1 hour.

2. Preheat the Air Fryer to 370 F. Roll each chunk in the crumb mixture. Place the crusted chicken in the fryer's basket. Spray with cooking spray. Cook for 8 minutes at 360 F, flipping once halfway through. Serve with a tomato dip or ketchup. Yum!

Cool Chicken Croquettes

Preparation Time: 20 min

Servings: 4

Nutrition Values: Calories: 230; Carbs: 10g; Fat: 12g; Protein: 9g

Ingredients

- 4 chicken breasts
- 1 whole egg
- Salt and pepper to taste
- 1 cup oats, crumbled
- ½ tsp garlic powder
- 1 tbsp parsley
- 1 tbsp thyme

Directions

1. Preheat your Air Fryer to 360 degrees F. Pulse chicken breast in a processor food until well blended. Add seasoning to the chicken alongside garlic, parsley, thyme

and mix well. In a bowl, add beaten egg and beat until the yolk is mixed.

2. In a separate bowl, add crumbled oats. Form croquettes using the chicken mixture and dip in beaten egg, and finally in oats until coated. Place the nuggets in your fryer's cooking basket. Cook for 10 minutes, making sure to keep shaking the basket after every 5 minutes.

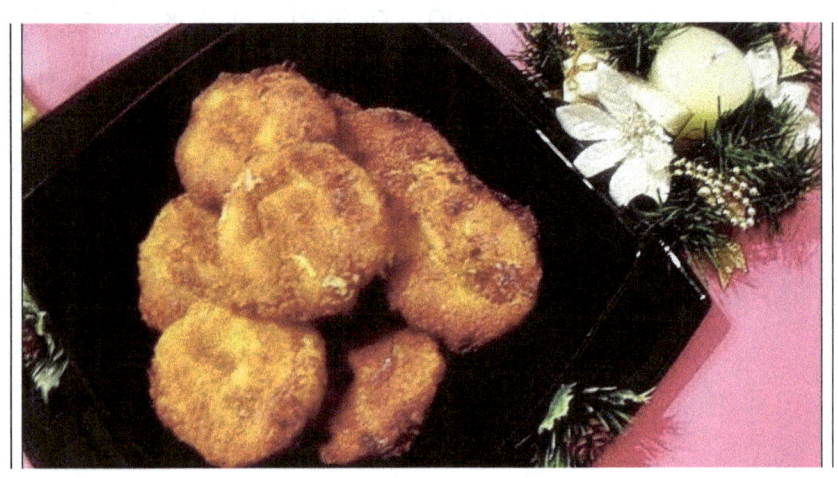

Herbed Croutons With Brie Cheese

Preparation Time: 20 min / Serve: 1

Nutrition Values: Calories: 20; Carbs: 1.5g; Fat: 1.3g; Protein: 0.5g

Ingredients

- 2 tbsp olive oil
- 1 tbsp french herbs
- 7 oz brie cheese, chopped
- 2 slices bread, halved

Directions

1. Preheat your Air Fryer to 340 degrees F. Using a bowl, mix oil with herbs. Dip the bread slices in the oil mixture to coat. Place the coated slices on a flat surface. Lay the brie cheese on the slices. Place the slices into your air fryer's basket and cook for 7 minutes. Once the bread is ready, cut into cubes.

Cheesy Bacon Fries

Preparation Time: 25 min

Servings: 4

Nutrition Values: Calories: 447; Carbs: 44g; Fat: 28g; Protein: 5g

Ingredients

- 2 large russet potatoes, cut strips
- 5 slices bacon, chopped
- 2 tbsp vegetable oil
- 2½ cups Cheddar cheese, shredded
- 3 oz melted cream cheese
- Salt and pepper to taste
- ¼ cup scallions, chopped

Directions

2. Boil salted water in a large sized pot. Add potatoes to the salted water and allow to boil for 4 minutes until blanched. Strain the potatoes in a colander and rinse thoroughly

with cold water to remove starch from the surface. Dry them with a kitchen towel. Preheat your Air Fryer to 400 F.

3. Add chopped bacon to your Air Fryer's cooking basket and cook for 4 minutes until crispy, making sure to give the basket a shake after 2 minutes; set aside. Add dried potatoes to the cooking basket and drizzle oil on top to coat. Cook for 25 minutes, shaking the basket every 5 minutes. Season with salt and pepper after 12 minutes.

4. Once cooked, transfer the fries to an 8-inch pan. In a bowl, mix 2 cups of cheddar cheese with cream cheese. Pour over the potatoes and add in crumbled bacon. Place the pan into the air fryer's cooking basket and cook for 5 more minutes at 340 F. Sprinkle chopped scallions on top and serve with your desired dressing.

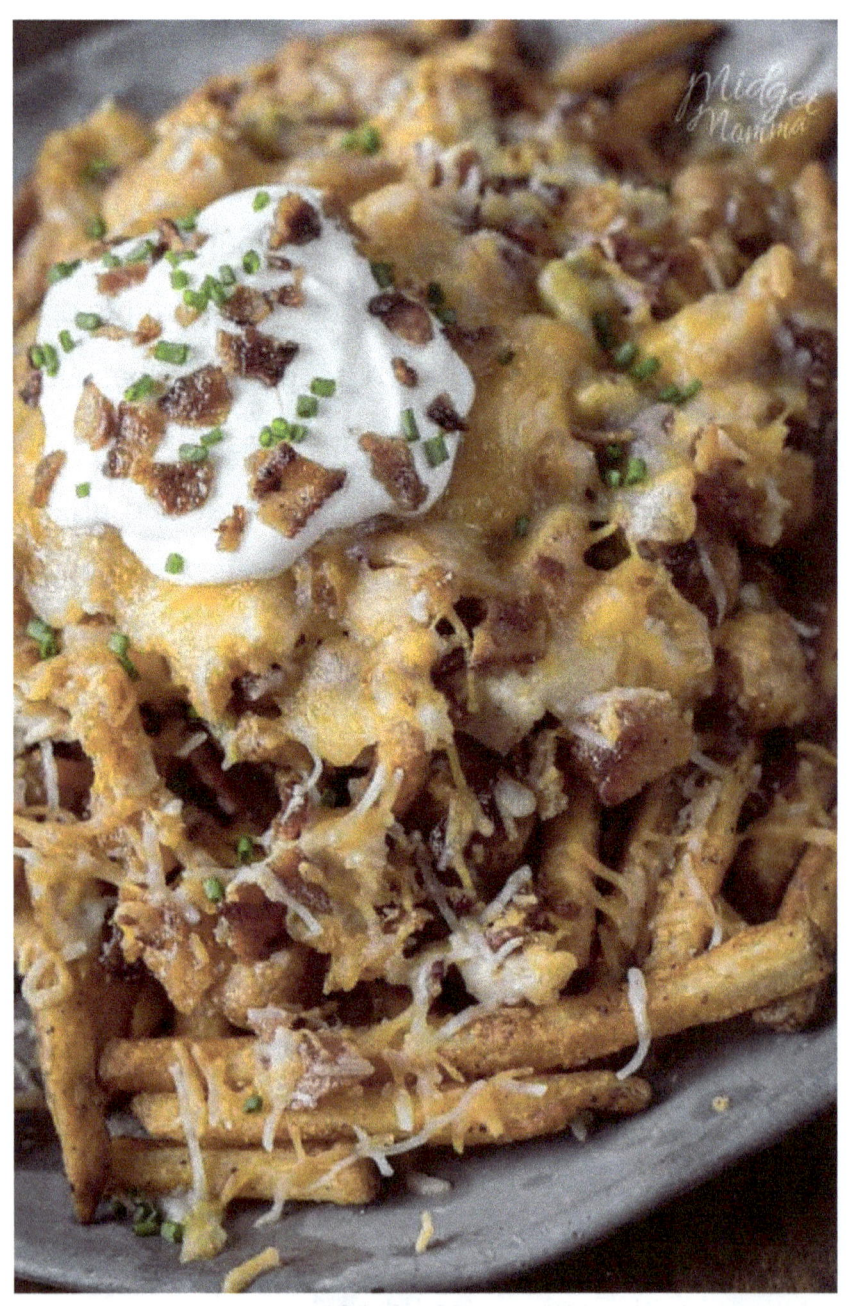

Oriental Grilled Family Steak

Servings: 3

Cooking Time: 50 minutes

Ingredients:

- 1/3 cup soy sauce
- 1/3 cup dry sherry
- 1 tablespoon brown sugar
- ½ teaspoon dry mustard
- 1 clove of garlic, minced
- 1 ½ pounds beef top round steak
- 2 green onions, chopped

Directions:

1. Place all ingredients except for the green onions in a Ziploc bag and allow to marinate in the fridge for at least 2 hours.

2. Preheat the air fryer at 3900F.

3. Place the grill pan accessory in the air fryer. Add meat and cover top with foil.
4. Grill for 50 minutes.
5. Halfway through the cooking time, flip the meat for even grilling.
6. Meanwhile, pour the marinade into a saucepan and simmer for 10 minutes until the sauce thickens.
7. Baste the meat with the sauce and garnish with green onions before serving.

Nutrition Values:

Calories: 170; Carbs: 3g; Protein: 28g; Fat: 5g

Tandoori Spiced Sirloin

Servings: 3

Cooking Time: 25 minutes

Ingredients:

- 1 ½ pounds boneless beef top loin steak
- ½ cup low-fat yogurt
- ¼ cup mint, chopped
- 3 tablespoons lemon juice
- 6 cloves of garlic, minced
- 2 teaspoons curry powder
- 2 teaspoons paprika
- Salt and pepper to taste

Directions:

1. Place all ingredients except for the green onions in a Ziploc bag and allow to marinate in the fridge for at least 2 hours.
2. Preheat the air fryer at 3900F.
3. Place the grill pan accessory in the air fryer.

4. Grill for 25 to 30 minutes.

5. Flip the steaks halfway through the cooking time for even grilling.

Nutrition Values:

Calories: 596; Carbs: 8.9g; Protein: 70.5g; Fat: 30.9g

Ribeye Steak with Peaches

Servings: 2

Cooking Time: 45 minutes

Ingredients:

- 1-pound T-bone steak
- 1 tablespoon paprika
- 2 teaspoons lemon pepper seasoning
- ¼ cup balsamic vinegar
- 1 cup peach puree
- Salt and pepper to taste
- 1 teaspoon thyme

Directions:

1. Place all ingredients in a Ziploc bag and allow to marinate in the fridge for at least 2 hours.
2. Preheat the air fryer at 3900F.
3. Place the grill pan accessory in the air fryer.

4. Grill for 20 minutes and flip the meat halfway through the cooking time.

Nutrition Values:

Calories: 570; Carbs: 35.7g; Protein: 47g; Fat: 26.5g

Kansas City Ribs

Servings: 2

Cooking Time: 50 minutes

Ingredients:

- 1-pound pork ribs, small
- 1 tablespoon brown sugar
- 1 teaspoon dry mustard
- ¼ teaspoon cayenne pepper
- 2 cloves of garlic
- 1 cup ketchup
- ¼ cup molasses
- ¼ cup apple cider vinegar
- 1 tablespoon Worcestershire sauce
- 1 tablespoon liquid smoke seasoning, hickory
- Salt and pepper to taste

Directions:

1. Place all ingredients in a Ziploc bag and allow to marinate in the fridge for at least 2 hours.
2. Preheat the air fryer at 3900F.
3. Place the grill pan accessory in the air fryer.
4. Grill meat for 25 minutes per batch.
5. Flip the meat halfway through the cooking time.
6. Pour the marinade in a saucepan and allow to simmer until the sauce thickens.
7. Pour glaze over the meat before serving.

Nutrition Values:

Calories: 634; Carbs: 32g; Protein: 32g; Fat: 42g

Grilled Steak Cubes with Charred Onions

Servings: 3

Cooking Time: 40 minutes

Ingredients:

- 1-pound boneless beef sirloin, cut into cubes
- 1 cup red onions, cut into wedges
- Salt and pepper to taste
- 1 tablespoon dry mustard
- 1 tablespoon olive oil

Directions:

1. Preheat the air fryer at 3900F.
2. Place the grill pan accessory in the air fryer.
3. Toss all ingredients in a bowl and mix until everything is coated with the seasonings.
4. Place on the grill pan and cook for 40 minutes.

5. Halfway through the cooking time, give a stir to cook evenly.

Nutrition Values:

Calories: 260; Carbs: 5.2g; Protein: 35.7g; Fat: 10.7g

Trip Tip Roast with Grilled Avocado

Servings: 4

Cooking Time: 50 minutes

Ingredients:

- 1 teaspoon onion powder
- 1 teaspoon garlic powder
- 1-pound beef tri-tip
- ½ cup red wine vinegar
- 3 tablespoons olive oil
- 3 avocadoes, seeded and sliced

Directions:

1. In a Ziploc bag, place all ingredients except for the avocado slices.
2. Allow to marinate in the fridge for 2 hours.
3. Preheat the air fryer at 3300F.
4. Place the grill pan accessory in the air fryer.

5. Grill the avocado for 2 minutes while the beef is marinating. Set aside.
6. After two hours, grill the beef for 50 minutes. Flip the beef halfway through the cooking time.
7. Serve the beef with grilled avocadoes

Nutrition Values:

Calories: 515; Carbs: 8g; Protein: 33g; Fat: 39g

Bourbon Grilled Beef

Servings: 4

Cooking Time: 60 minutes

Ingredients:

- 2 pounds beef steak, pounded
- ¼ cup bourbon
- ¼ cup barbecue sauce
- 1 tablespoon Worcestershire sauce
- Salt and pepper to taste

Directions:

1. Place all ingredients in a Ziploc bag and allow to marinate in the fridge for at least 2 hours.
2. Preheat the air fryer at 3900F.
3. Place the grill pan accessory in the air fryer.
4. Place on the grill pan and cook for 20 minutes per batch.

5. Halfway through the cooking time, give a stir to cook evenly.
6. Meanwhile, pour the marinade on a saucepan and allow to simmer until the sauce thickens.
7. Serve beef with the bourbon sauce.

Nutrition Values:

Calories: 346; Carbs: 9.8g; Protein: 48.2g; Fat: 12.6g

Paprika Beef Flank Steak

Servings: 4

Cooking Time: 40 minutes

Ingredients:

- 1 ¼ pounds beef flank steak, sliced thinly
- Salt and pepper to taste
- 3 tablespoons paprika powder
- 1 tablespoon cayenne pepper
- 1 tablespoon garlic powder
- 1 tablespoon onion powder
- 1 red bell pepper, julienned
- 1 yellow bell pepper, julienned
- 3 tablespoons olive oil

Directions:

1. Preheat the air fryer at 3900F.
2. Place the grill pan accessory in the air fryer.
3. In a bowl, toss all ingredients to coat everything with the seasonings.

4. Place on the grill pan and cook for 40 minutes.
5. Make sure to stir every 10 minutes for even cooking.

Nutrition Values:

Calories: 334; Carbs: 9.8g; Protein: 32.5g; Fat: 18.2g

Espresso-Rubbed Steak

Servings: 3

Cooking Time: 50 minutes

Ingredients:

- 2 teaspoons chili powder
- Salt and pepper to taste
- 1 teaspoon instant espresso powder
- ½ teaspoon garlic powder
- 1 ½ pounds beef flank steak
- 2 tablespoons olive oil

Directions:

1. Preheat the air fryer at 3900F.
2. Place the grill pan accessory in the air fryer.
3. Make the dry rub by mixing the chili powder, salt, pepper, espresso powder, and garlic powder.
4. Rub all over the steak and brush with oil.

5. Place on the grill pan and cook for 40 minutes.
6. Halfway through the cooking time, flip the beef to cook evenly.

Nutrition Values:

Calories: 249; Carbs: 4g; Protein: 20g; Fat: 17g

New York Beef Strips

Servings: 4

Cooking Time: 50 minutes

Ingredients:

- 4 boneless beef top loin steaks
- Salt and pepper to taste
- 2 tablespoons butter, softened
- 2 pounds crumbled blue cheese
- 2 tablespoons cream cheese
- 1 tablespoon pine nuts, toasted

Directions:

1. Preheat the air fryer at 3900F.
2. Place the grill pan accessory in the air fryer.
3. Season the beef with salt and pepper. Brush all sides with butter.
4. Grill for 25 minutes per batch making sure to flip halfway through the cooking time.

5. Slice the beef and serve with blue cheese, cream cheese and pine nuts.

Nutrition Values:

Calories: 682; Carbs: 1g; Protein: 75g; Fat: 42g

Perfect Yet Simple Grilled Steak

Servings: 2

Cooking Time: 50 minutes

Ingredients:

- 2 large ribeye strip steaks
- Salt and pepper to taste
- 1 teaspoon liquid smoke seasoning, hickory

Directions:

1. Preheat the air fryer at 3900F.
2. Place the grill pan accessory in the air fryer.
3. Season the beef with salt, pepper, and liquid seasoning.
4. Grill for 25 minutes per batch.
5. Flip the meat halfway through the cooking time for even browning.

Nutrition Values:

Calories: 476; Carbs: 7g; Protein: 49g; Fat: 28g

Smoked Beef Chuck

Servings: 6

Cooking Time: 1 hour and 30 minutes

Ingredients:

- 3 pounds beef chuck roll, scored with knife
- 2 ounces black peppercorns
- 3 tablespoons salt
- 2 tablespoons olive oil

Directions:

1. Preheat the air fryer at 3900F.
2. Place the grill pan accessory in the air fryer.
3. Season the beef chuck roll with black peppercorns and salt.
4. Brush with olive oil and cover top with foil.
5. Grill for 1 hour and 30 minutes.
6. Flip the beef every 30 minutes for even grilling on all sides.

Nutrition Values:

Calories: 360; Carbs: 1.4g; Protein: 46.7g; Fat: 18g

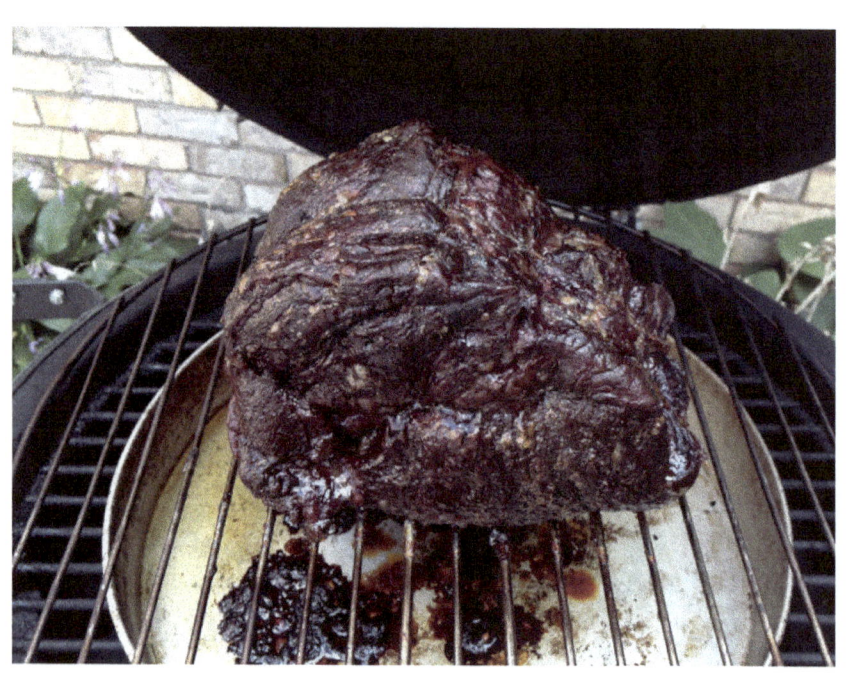

Sous Vide Smoked Brisket

Servings: 6

Cooking Time: 1 hour

Ingredients:

- 3 pounds flat-cut brisket
- ¼ teaspoon liquid smoke
- Salt and pepper to taste
- 1 cup dill pickles

Directions:

1. Preheat the air fryer at 3900F.
2. Place the grill pan accessory in the air fryer.
3. Season the brisket with liquid smoke, salt, and pepper.
4. Place on the grill pan and cook for 30 minutes per batch.
5. Flip the meat halfway through cooking time for even grilling.
6. Serve with dill pickles.

Nutrition Values:

Calories: 309; Carbs: 1.2g; Protein: 49g; Fat:12 g

Skirt Steak with Mojo Marinade

Servings: 4

Cooking Time: 60 minutes

Ingredients:

- 2 pounds skirt steak, trimmed from excess fat
- 2 tablespoons lime juice
- ¼ cup orange juice
- 2 tablespoons olive oil
- 4 cloves of garlic, minced
- 1 teaspoon ground cumin
- Salt and pepper to taste

Directions:

1. Place all ingredients in a mixing bowl and allow to marinate in the fridge for at least 2 hours
2. Preheat the air fryer at 3900F.

3. Place the grill pan accessory in the air fryer.
4. Grill for 15 minutes per batch and flip the beef every 8 minutes for even grilling.
5. Meanwhile, pour the marinade on a saucepan and allow to simmer for 10 minutes or until the sauce thickens.
6. Slice the beef and pour over the sauce.

Nutrition Values:

Calories: 568; Carbs: 4.7g; Protein: 59.1g; Fat: 34.7g

Dijon-Marinated Skirt Steak

Servings: 2

Cooking Time: 40 minutes

Ingredients:

- ¼ cup Dijon mustard
- 1-pound skirt steak, trimmed
- 2 tablespoons champagne vinegar
- 1 tablespoon rosemary leaves
- Salt and pepper to taste

Directions:

1. Place all ingredients in a Ziploc bag and marinate in the fridge for 2 hours.
2. Preheat the air fryer at 3900F.
3. Place the grill pan accessory in the air fryer.
4. Grill the skirt steak for 20 minutes per batch.
5. Flip the beef halfway through the cooking time.

Nutrition Values:

Calories: 516; Carbs: 4.2g; Protein: 60.9g; Fat: 28.4g

Grilled Carne Asada Steak

Servings: 2

Cooking Time: 50 minutes

Ingredients:

- 2 slices skirt steak
- 1 dried ancho chilies, chopped
- 1 chipotle pepper, chopped
- 2 tablespoons of fresh lemon juice
- 2 tablespoons olive oil
- 3 cloves of garlic, minced
- 1 tablespoons soy sauce
- 2 tablespoons Asian fish sauce
- 1 tablespoon cumin
- 1 tablespoon coriander seeds
- 2 tablespoons brown sugar

Directions:

1. Place all ingredients in a Ziploc bag and marinate in the fridge for 2 hours.

2. Preheat the air fryer at 3900F.

3. Place the grill pan accessory in the air fryer.

4. Grill the skirt steak for 20 minutes.

5. Flip the steak every 10 minutes for even grilling.

Nutrition Values:

Calories: 697; Carbs: 10.2g; Protein:62.7 g; Fat: 45g

Chimichurri-Style Steak

Servings: 6

Cooking Time: 60 minutes

Ingredients:

- 3 pounds steak
- Salt and pepper to taste
- 1 cup commercial chimichurri

Directions:

1. Place all ingredients in a Ziploc bag and marinate in the fridge for 2 hours.
2. Preheat the air fryer at 3900F.
3. Place the grill pan accessory in the air fryer.
4. Grill the skirt steak for 20 minutes per batch.
5. Flip the steak every 10 minutes for even grilling.

Nutrition Values:

Calories: 507; Carbs: 2.8g; Protein: 63g; Fat: 27g

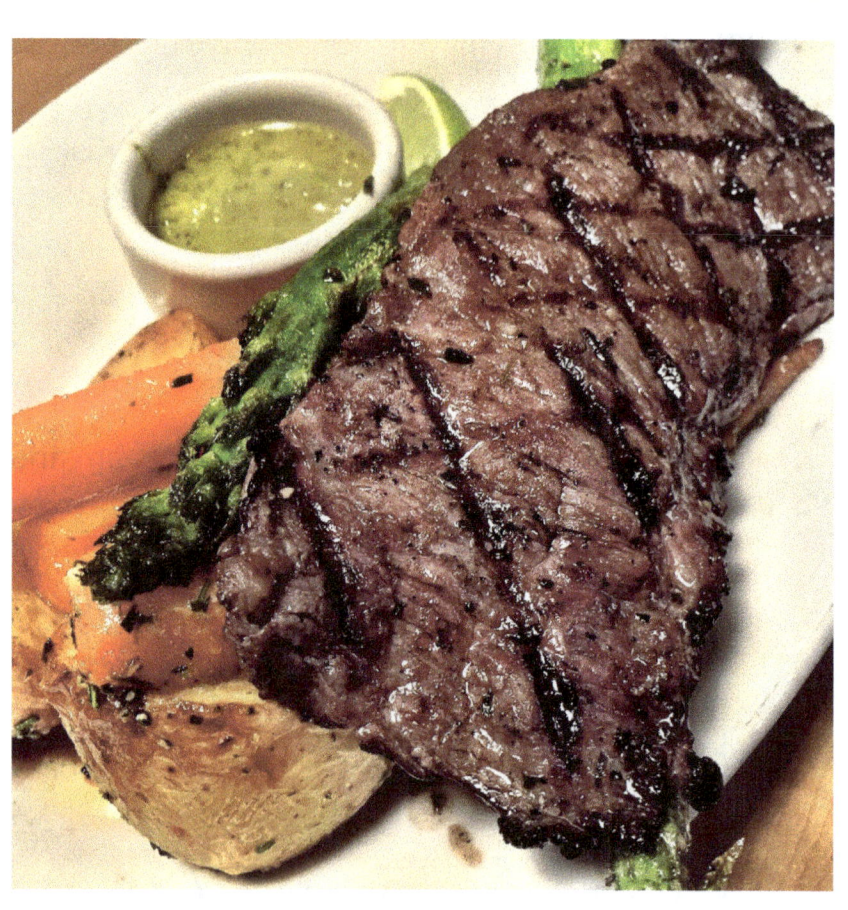

Strip Steak with Cucumber Yogurt Sauce

Servings: 2

Cooking Time: 50 minutes

Ingredients:

- 2 New York strip steaks
- Salt and pepper to taste
- 3 tablespoons olive oil
- 1 cucumber, seeded and chopped
- 1 cup Greek yogurt
- ½ cup parsley, chopped

Directions:

1. Preheat the air fryer at 3900F.
2. Place the grill pan accessory in the air fryer.
3. Season the strip steaks with salt and pepper. Drizzle with oil.

4. Grill the steak for 20 minutes per batch and make sure to flip the meat every 10 minutes for even grilling.
5. Meanwhile, combine the cucumber, yogurt, and parsley.
6. Serve the beef with the cucumber yogurt.

Nutrition Values:

Calories: 460; Carbs: 5.2g; Protein: 50.8g; Fat: 26.3g

Pork Bites

Preparation time: 10 minutes

Cooking time: 15 minutes

Servings: 4

Ingredients:

- 2 teaspoons garlic powder
- 2 eggs
- Salt and black pepper to taste
- ¾ cup panko breadcrumbs
- ¾ cup coconut, shredded
- A drizzle of olive oil
- 1 pound ground pork

Directions:

1. In a bowl, mix coconut with panko and stir well.
2. In another bowl, mix the pork, salt, pepper, eggs, and garlic powder, and then shape medium meatballs out of this mix.

3. Dredge the meatballs in the coconut mix, place them in your air fryer's basket, introduce in the air fryer, and cook at 350 degrees F for 15 minutes.
4. Serve and enjoy!

Nutrition Values: calories 192, fat 4, fiber 2, carbs 14, protein 6

Banana Chips

Preparation time: 5 minutes

Cooking time: 5 minutes

Servings: 8

Ingredients:

- ¼ cup peanut butter, soft
- 1 banana, peeled and sliced into 16 pieces
- 1 tablespoon vegetable oil

Directions:

1. Put the banana slices in your air fryer's basket and drizzle the oil over them.
2. Cook at 360 degrees F for 5 minutes.
3. Transfer to bowls and serve them dipped in peanut butter.

Nutrition Values: calories 100, fat 4, fiber 1, carbs 10, protein 4

Lemony Apple Bites

Preparation time: 5 minutes

Cooking time: 5 minutes

Servings: 4

Ingredients:

- 3 big apples, cored, peeled and cubed
- 2 teaspoons lemon juice
- ½ cup caramel sauce

Directions:

1. In your air fryer, mix all the ingredients; toss well.
2. Cook at 340 degrees F for 5 minutes.
3. Divide into cups and serve as a snack.

Nutrition Values: calories 180, fat 4, fiber 3, carbs 10, protein 3

Zucchini Balls

Preparation time: 10 minutes

Cooking time: 12 minutes

Servings: 8

Ingredients:

- Cooking spray
- ½ cup dill, chopped
- 1 egg
- ½ cup white flour
- Salt and black pepper to taste
- 2 garlic cloves, minced
- 3 zucchinis, grated

Directions:

1. In a bowl, mix all the ingredients and stir.
2. Shape the mix into medium balls and place them into your air fryer's basket.
3. Cook at 375 degrees F for 12 minutes, flipping them halfway.

4. Serve them as a snack right away.

Nutrition Values: calories 120, fat 1, fiber 2, carbs 5, protein 3

Basil and Cilantro Crackers

Preparation time: 10 minutes

Cooking time: 16 minutes

Servings: 6

Ingredients:

- ½ teaspoon baking powder
- Salt and black pepper to taste
- 1¼ cups flour
- 1 garlic clove, minced
- 2 tablespoons basil, minced
- 2 tablespoons cilantro, minced
- 4 tablespoons butter, melted

Directions:

1. Add all of the ingredients to a bowl and stir until you obtain a dough.
2. Spread this on a lined baking sheet that fits your air fryer.

3. Place the baking sheet in the fryer at 325 degrees F and cook for 16 minutes.

4. Cool down, cut, and serve.

Nutrition Values: calories 171, fat 9, fiber 1, carbs 8, protein 4

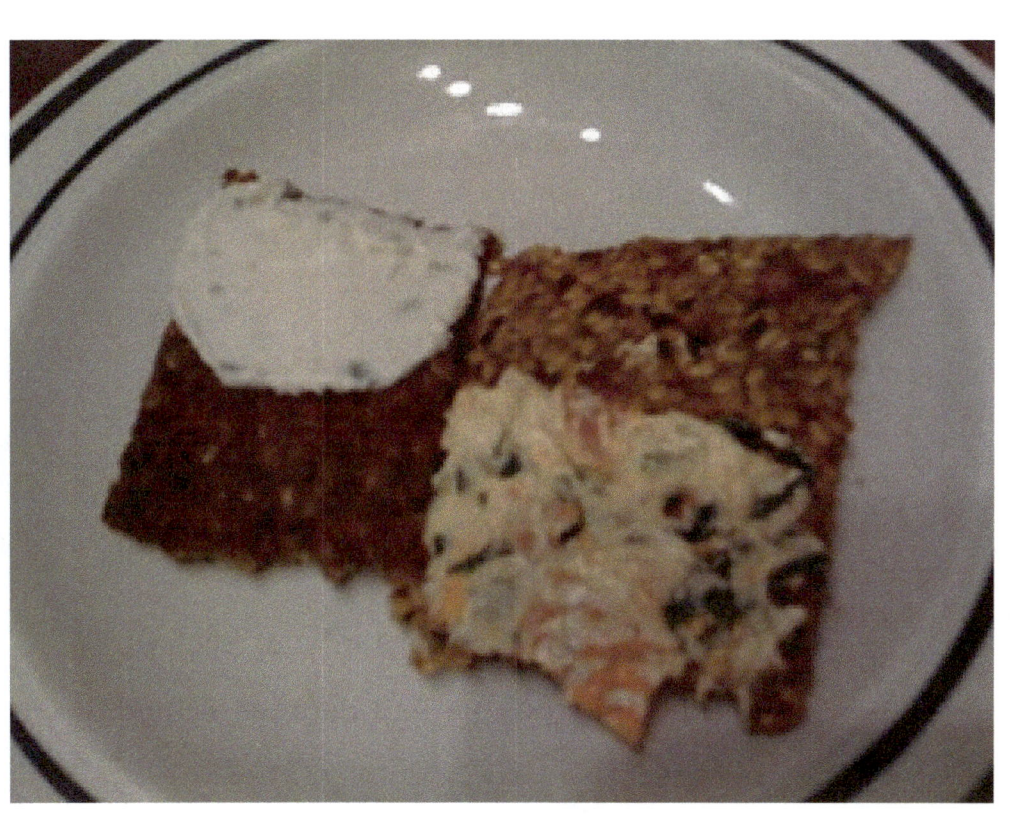

Balsamic Zucchini Slices

Preparation time: 5 minutes

Cooking time: 50 minutes

Servings: 6

Ingredients:

- 3 zucchinis, thinly sliced
- Salt and black pepper to taste
- 2 tablespoons avocado oil
- 2 tablespoons balsamic vinegar

Directions:

1. Add all of the ingredients to a bowl and mix.
2. Put the zucchini mixture in your air fryer's basket and cook at 220 degrees F for 50 minutes.
3. Serve as a snack and enjoy!

Nutrition Values: calories 40, fat 3, fiber 7, carbs 3, protein 7

Turmeric Carrot Chips

Preparation time: 5 minutes

Cooking time: 25 minutes

Servings: 4

Ingredients:

- 4 carrots, thinly sliced
- Salt and black pepper to taste
- ½ teaspoon turmeric powder
- ½ teaspoon chaat masala
- 1 teaspoon olive oil

Directions:

1. Place all ingredients in a bowl and toss well.
2. Put the mixture in your air fryer's basket and cook at 370 degrees F for 25 minutes, shaking the fryer from time to time.
3. Serve as a snack.

Nutrition Values: calories 161, fat 1, fiber 2, carbs 5, protein 3

Chives Radish Snack

Preparation time: 5 minutes

Cooking time: 10 minutes

Servings: 4

Ingredients:

- 16 radishes, sliced
- A drizzle of olive oil
- Salt and black pepper to taste
- 1 tablespoon chives, chopped

Directions:

1. In a bowl, mix the radishes, salt, pepper, and oil; toss well.
2. Place the radishes in your air fryer's basket and cook at 350 degrees F for 10 minutes.
3. Divide into bowls and serve with chives sprinkled on top.

Nutrition Values: calories 100, fat 1, fiber 2, carbs 4, protein 1

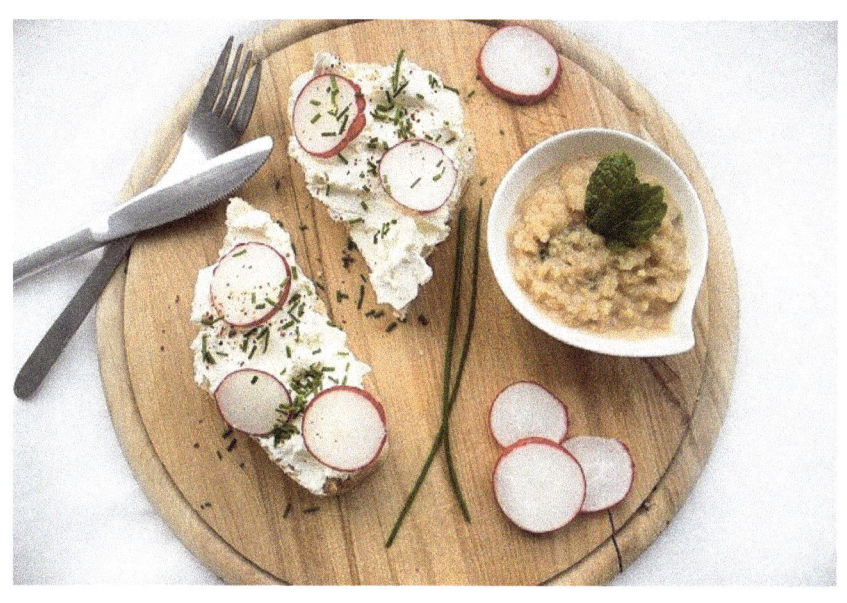

www.ingramcontent.com/pod-product-compliance
Lightning Source LLC
Chambersburg PA
CBHW070725030426
42336CB00013B/1915